Daycare

Medication

Log

Table of Contents

CHILD'S NAME	PAGE NUMBER
	4-5
	6-7
	8-9
	10-11
	12-13
	14-15
	16-17
	18-19
	20-21
	22-23
	24-25
	26-27
	28-29
	30-31
	32-33
	34-35
	36-37
	38-39
	40-41
	42-43
	44-45
	46-47
	48-49
	50-51
	52-53

Medication Authorization and Instructions

Child's Name _____

Date _____

I grant permission to my childcare provider, _____
to administer the following medication to my child. I will therefore not hold my childcare provider liable in the event of reactions or complications arising from my child receiving this medication, once same is administered as per my instructions below.

Parent's signature _____

Instructions Log							
Date	Medication	Start Date	Finish Date	Dosage	Time	Parent's Signature	Administrator's Signature

		Instructions Log						
Date	Medication	Start Date	Finish Date	Dosage	Time	Parent's Signature	Administrator's Signature

Medication Authorization and Instructions

Child's Name _____

Date _____

I grant permission to my childcare provider, _____
to administer the following medication to my child. I will therefore not hold my
childcare provider liable in the event of reactions or complications arising from
my child receiving this medication, once same is administered as per my
instructions below.

Parent's signature _____

Instructions Log							
Date	Medication	Start Date	Finish Date	Dosage	Time	Parent's Signature	Administrator's Signature

		Instructions Log					
Date	Medication	Start Date	Finish Date	Dosage	Time	Parent's Signature	Administrator's Signature

Medication Authorization and Instructions

Child's Name _____

Date _____

I grant permission to my childcare provider, _____
to administer the following medication to my child. I will therefore not hold my
childcare provider liable in the event of reactions or complications arising from
my child receiving this medication, once same is administered as per my
instructions below.

Parent's signature _____

Instructions Log							
Date	Medication	Start Date	Finish Date	Dosage	Time	Parent's Signature	Administrator's Signature

		Instructions Log						
Date	Medication	Start Date	Finish Date	Dosage	Time	Parent's Signature	Administrator's Signature

Medication Authorization and Instructions

Child's Name _____

Date _____

I grant permission to my childcare provider, _____
to administer the following medication to my child. I will therefore not hold my childcare provider liable in the event of reactions or complications arising from my child receiving this medication, once same is administered as per my instructions below.

Parent's signature _____

Instructions Log							
Date	Medication	Start Date	Finish Date	Dosage	Time	Parent's Signature	Administrator's Signature

Date	Medication	Start Date	Finish Date	Dosage	Time	Parent's Signature	Administrator's Signature

Instructions Log

Medication Authorization and Instructions

Child's Name _____

Date _____

I grant permission to my childcare provider, _____
to administer the following medication to my child. I will therefore not hold my childcare provider liable in the event of reactions or complications arising from my child receiving this medication, once same is administered as per my instructions below.

Parent's signature _____

Instructions Log							
Date	Medication	Start Date	Finish Date	Dosage	Time	Parent's Signature	Administrator's Signature

Instructions Log							
Date	Medication	Start Date	Finish Date	Dosage	Time	Parent's Signature	Administrator's Signature

Medication Authorization and Instructions

Child's Name _____

Date _____

I grant permission to my childcare provider, _____
to administer the following medication to my child. I will therefore not hold my
childcare provider liable in the event of reactions or complications arising from
my child receiving this medication, once same is administered as per my
instructions below.

Parent's signature _____

Instructions Log							
Date	Medication	Start Date	Finish Date	Dosage	Time	Parent's Signature	Administrator's Signature

Date	Medication	Start Date	Finish Date	Dosage	Time	Parent's Signature	Administrator's Signature

Medication Authorization and Instructions

Child's Name _____

Date _____

I grant permission to my childcare provider, _____
to administer the following medication to my child. I will therefore not hold my childcare provider liable in the event of reactions or complications arising from my child receiving this medication, once same is administered as per my instructions below.

Parent's signature _____

Instructions Log							
Date	Medication	Start Date	Finish Date	Dosage	Time	Parent's Signature	Administrator's Signature

Instructions Log							
Date	Medication	Start Date	Finish Date	Dosage	Time	Parent's Signature	Administrator's Signature

Medication Authorization and Instructions

Child's Name _____

Date _____

I grant permission to my childcare provider, _____
to administer the following medication to my child. I will therefore not hold my
childcare provider liable in the event of reactions or complications arising from
my child receiving this medication, once same is administered as per my
instructions below.

Parent's signature _____

Instructions Log							
Date	Medication	Start Date	Finish Date	Dosage	Time	Parent's Signature	Administrator's Signature

Date	Medication	Start Date	Finish Date	Dosage	Time	Parent's Signature	Administrator's Signature

Instructions Log

Medication Authorization and Instructions

Child's Name _____

Date _____

I grant permission to my childcare provider, _____
to administer the following medication to my child. I will therefore not hold my
childcare provider liable in the event of reactions or complications arising from
my child receiving this medication, once same is administered as per my
instructions below.

Parent's signature _____

Instructions Log							
Date	Medication	Start Date	Finish Date	Dosage	Time	Parent's Signature	Administrator's Signature

		Instructions Log						
Date	Medication	Start Date	Finish Date	Dosage	Time	Parent's Signature	Administrator's Signature

Medication Authorization and Instructions

Child's Name _____

Date _____

I grant permission to my childcare provider, _____
to administer the following medication to my child. I will therefore not hold my childcare provider liable in the event of reactions or complications arising from my child receiving this medication, once same is administered as per my instructions below.

Parent's signature _____

Instructions Log							
Date	Medication	Start Date	Finish Date	Dosage	Time	Parent's Signature	Administrator's Signature

Date	Medication	Start Date	Finish Date	Dosage	Time	Parent's Signature	Administrator's Signature

Instructions Log

Medication Authorization and Instructions

Child's Name _____

Date _____

I grant permission to my childcare provider, _____
to administer the following medication to my child. I will therefore not hold my childcare provider liable in the event of reactions or complications arising from my child receiving this medication, once same is administered as per my instructions below.

Parent's signature _____

Instructions Log							
Date	Medication	Start Date	Finish Date	Dosage	Time	Parent's Signature	Administrator's Signature

Date	Medication	Start Date	Finish Date	Dosage	Time	Parent's Signature	Administrator's Signature

Instructions Log

Medication Authorization and Instructions

Child's Name _____

Date _____

I grant permission to my childcare provider, _____
to administer the following medication to my child. I will therefore not hold my
childcare provider liable in the event of reactions or complications arising from
my child receiving this medication, once same is administered as per my
instructions below.

Parent's signature _____

Instructions Log							
Date	Medication	Start Date	Finish Date	Dosage	Time	Parent's Signature	Administrator's Signature

Date	Medication	Start Date	Finish Date	Dosage	Time	Parent's Signature	Administrator's Signature

Instructions Log

Medication Authorization and Instructions

Child's Name _____

Date _____

I grant permission to my childcare provider, _____
to administer the following medication to my child. I will therefore not hold my childcare provider liable in the event of reactions or complications arising from my child receiving this medication, once same is administered as per my instructions below.

Parent's signature _____

Instructions Log							
Date	Medication	Start Date	Finish Date	Dosage	Time	Parent's Signature	Administrator's Signature

Date	Medication	Start Date	Finish Date	Dosage	Time	Parent's Signature	Administrator's Signature

Instructions Log

Medication Authorization and Instructions

Child's Name _____

Date _____

I grant permission to my childcare provider, _____
to administer the following medication to my child. I will therefore not hold my
childcare provider liable in the event of reactions or complications arising from
my child receiving this medication, once same is administered as per my
instructions below.

Parent's signature _____

Instructions Log							
Date	Medication	Start Date	Finish Date	Dosage	Time	Parent's Signature	Administrator's Signature

Date	Medication	Start Date	Finish Date	Dosage	Time	Parent's Signature	Administrator's Signature

Instructions Log

Medication Authorization and Instructions

Child's Name _____

Date _____

I grant permission to my childcare provider, _____
to administer the following medication to my child. I will therefore not hold my
childcare provider liable in the event of reactions or complications arising from
my child receiving this medication, once same is administered as per my
instructions below.

Parent's signature _____

Instructions Log							
Date	Medication	Start Date	Finish Date	Dosage	Time	Parent's Signature	Administrator's Signature

Date	Medication	Start Date	Finish Date	Dosage	Time	Parent's Signature	Administrator's Signature

Instructions Log

Medication Authorization and Instructions

Child's Name _____

Date _____

I grant permission to my childcare provider, _____
to administer the following medication to my child. I will therefore not hold my childcare provider liable in the event of reactions or complications arising from my child receiving this medication, once same is administered as per my instructions below.

Parent's signature _____

Instructions Log							
Date	Medication	Start Date	Finish Date	Dosage	Time	Parent's Signature	Administrator's Signature

		Instructions Log					
Date	Medication	Start Date	Finish Date	Dosage	Time	Parent's Signature	Administrator's Signature

Medication Authorization and Instructions

Child's Name _____

Date _____

I grant permission to my childcare provider, _____
to administer the following medication to my child. I will therefore not hold my childcare provider liable in the event of reactions or complications arising from my child receiving this medication, once same is administered as per my instructions below.

Parent's signature _____

Instructions Log							
Date	Medication	Start Date	Finish Date	Dosage	Time	Parent's Signature	Administrator's Signature

Date	Medication	Start Date	Finish Date	Dosage	Time	Parent's Signature	Administrator's Signature

Instructions Log

Medication Authorization and Instructions

Child's Name _____

Date _____

I grant permission to my childcare provider, _____
to administer the following medication to my child. I will therefore not hold my childcare provider liable in the event of reactions or complications arising from my child receiving this medication, once same is administered as per my instructions below.

Parent's signature _____

Instructions Log							
Date	Medication	Start Date	Finish Date	Dosage	Time	Parent's Signature	Administrator's Signature

		Instructions Log						
Date	Medication	Start Date	Finish Date	Dosage	Time	Parent's Signature	Administrator's Signature

Medication Authorization and Instructions

Child's Name _____

Date _____

I grant permission to my childcare provider, _____
to administer the following medication to my child. I will therefore not hold my childcare provider liable in the event of reactions or complications arising from my child receiving this medication, once same is administered as per my instructions below.

Parent's signature _____

Instructions Log							
Date	Medication	Start Date	Finish Date	Dosage	Time	Parent's Signature	Administrator's Signature

Date	Medication	Start Date	Finish Date	Dosage	Time	Parent's Signature	Administrator's Signature

Medication Authorization and Instructions

Child's Name _____

Date _____

I grant permission to my childcare provider, _____
to administer the following medication to my child. I will therefore not hold my childcare provider liable in the event of reactions or complications arising from my child receiving this medication, once same is administered as per my instructions below.

Parent's signature _____

Instructions Log							
Date	Medication	Start Date	Finish Date	Dosage	Time	Parent's Signature	Administrator's Signature

Date	Medication	Start Date	Finish Date	Dosage	Time	Parent's Signature	Administrator's Signature

Medication Authorization and Instructions

Child's Name _____

Date _____

I grant permission to my childcare provider, _____
to administer the following medication to my child. I will therefore not hold my
childcare provider liable in the event of reactions or complications arising from
my child receiving this medication, once same is administered as per my
instructions below.

Parent's signature _____

Instructions Log							
Date	Medication	Start Date	Finish Date	Dosage	Time	Parent's Signature	Administrator's Signature

Date	Medication	Start Date	Finish Date	Dosage	Time	Parent's Signature	Administrator's Signature

Medication Authorization and Instructions

Child's Name _____

Date _____

I grant permission to my childcare provider, _____
to administer the following medication to my child. I will therefore not hold my childcare provider liable in the event of reactions or complications arising from my child receiving this medication, once same is administered as per my instructions below.

Parent's signature _____

Instructions Log							
Date	Medication	Start Date	Finish Date	Dosage	Time	Parent's Signature	Administrator's Signature

		Instructions Log					
Date	Medication	Start Date	Finish Date	Dosage	Time	Parent's Signature	Administrator's Signature

Medication Authorization and Instructions

Child's Name _____

Date _____

I grant permission to my childcare provider, _____
to administer the following medication to my child. I will therefore not hold my
childcare provider liable in the event of reactions or complications arising from
my child receiving this medication, once same is administered as per my
instructions below.

Parent's signature _____

Instructions Log							
Date	Medication	Start Date	Finish Date	Dosage	Time	Parent's Signature	Administrator's Signature

Date	Medication	Start Date	Finish Date	Dosage	Time	Parent's Signature	Administrator's Signature

Instructions Log

Medication Authorization and Instructions

Child's Name _____

Date _____

I grant permission to my childcare provider, _____
to administer the following medication to my child. I will therefore not hold my childcare provider liable in the event of reactions or complications arising from my child receiving this medication, once same is administered as per my instructions below.

Parent's signature _____

Instructions Log							
Date	Medication	Start Date	Finish Date	Dosage	Time	Parent's Signature	Administrator's Signature

		Instructions Log						
Date	Medication	Start Date	Finish Date	Dosage	Time	Parent's Signature	Administrator's Signature

Medication Authorization and Instructions

Child's Name _____

Date _____

I grant permission to my childcare provider, _____
to administer the following medication to my child. I will therefore not hold my childcare provider liable in the event of reactions or complications arising from my child receiving this medication, once same is administered as per my instructions below.

Parent's signature _____

Instructions Log							
Date	Medication	Start Date	Finish Date	Dosage	Time	Parent's Signature	Administrator's Signature

Date	Medication	Start Date	Finish Date	Dosage	Time	Parent's Signature	Administrator's Signature

Instructions Log

Medication Authorization and Instructions

Child's Name _____

Date _____

I grant permission to my childcare provider, _____
to administer the following medication to my child. I will therefore not hold my childcare provider liable in the event of reactions or complications arising from my child receiving this medication, once same is administered as per my instructions below.

Parent's signature _____

Instructions Log							
Date	Medication	Start Date	Finish Date	Dosage	Time	Parent's Signature	Administrator's Signature

Date	Medication	Start Date	Finish Date	Dosage	Time	Parent's Signature	Administrator's Signature

Medication Authorization and Instructions

Child's Name _____

Date _____

I grant permission to my childcare provider, _____
to administer the following medication to my child. I will therefore not hold my childcare provider liable in the event of reactions or complications arising from my child receiving this medication, once same is administered as per my instructions below.

Parent's signature _____

Instructions Log							
Date	Medication	Start Date	Finish Date	Dosage	Time	Parent's Signature	Administrator's Signature

Date	Medication	Start Date	Finish Date	Dosage	Time	Parent's Signature	Administrator's Signature

Instructions Log

Medication Authorization and Instructions

Child's Name _____

Date _____

I grant permission to my childcare provider, _____
to administer the following medication to my child. I will therefore not hold my childcare provider liable in the event of reactions or complications arising from my child receiving this medication, once same is administered as per my instructions below.

Parent's signature _____

Instructions Log							
Date	Medication	Start Date	Finish Date	Dosage	Time	Parent's Signature	Administrator's Signature

					Instructions Log		
Date	Medication	Start Date	Finish Date	Dosage	Time	Parent's Signature	Administrator's Signature

Medication Authorization and Instructions

Child's Name _____

Date _____

I grant permission to my childcare provider, _____
to administer the following medication to my child. I will therefore not hold my
childcare provider liable in the event of reactions or complications arising from
my child receiving this medication, once same is administered as per my
instructions below.

Parent's signature _____

Instructions Log							
Date	Medication	Start Date	Finish Date	Dosage	Time	Parent's Signature	Administrator's Signature

Date	Medication	Start Date	Finish Date	Dosage	Time	Parent's Signature	Administrator's Signature

Instructions Log

Medication Authorization and Instructions

Child's Name _____

Date _____

I grant permission to my childcare provider, _____
to administer the following medication to my child. I will therefore not hold my childcare provider liable in the event of reactions or complications arising from my child receiving this medication, once same is administered as per my instructions below.

Parent's signature _____

Instructions Log							
Date	Medication	Start Date	Finish Date	Dosage	Time	Parent's Signature	Administrator's Signature

Instructions Log

Date	Medication	Start Date	Finish Date	Dosage	Time	Parent's Signature	Administrator's Signature

Medication Authorization and Instructions

Child's Name _____

Date _____

I grant permission to my childcare provider, _____
to administer the following medication to my child. I will therefore not hold my
childcare provider liable in the event of reactions or complications arising from
my child receiving this medication, once same is administered as per my
instructions below.

Parent's signature _____

Instructions Log							
Date	Medication	Start Date	Finish Date	Dosage	Time	Parent's Signature	Administrator's Signature

Date	Medication	Start Date	Finish Date	Dosage	Time	Parent's Signature	Administrator's Signature

Medication Authorization and Instructions

Child's Name _____

Date _____

I grant permission to my childcare provider, _____
to administer the following medication to my child. I will therefore not hold my childcare provider liable in the event of reactions or complications arising from my child receiving this medication, once same is administered as per my instructions below.

Parent's signature _____

Instructions Log							
Date	Medication	Start Date	Finish Date	Dosage	Time	Parent's Signature	Administrator's Signature

		Instructions Log					
Date	Medication	Start Date	Finish Date	Dosage	Time	Parent's Signature	Administrator's Signature

Medication Authorization and Instructions

Child's Name _____

Date _____

I grant permission to my childcare provider, _____
to administer the following medication to my child. I will therefore not hold my childcare provider liable in the event of reactions or complications arising from my child receiving this medication, once same is administered as per my instructions below.

Parent's signature _____

Instructions Log							
Date	Medication	Start Date	Finish Date	Dosage	Time	Parent's Signature	Administrator's Signature

Date	Medication	Start Date	Finish Date	Dosage	Time	Parent's Signature	Administrator's Signature

Instructions Log

Medication Authorization and Instructions

Child's Name _____

Date _____

I grant permission to my childcare provider, _____
to administer the following medication to my child. I will therefore not hold my childcare provider liable in the event of reactions or complications arising from my child receiving this medication, once same is administered as per my instructions below.

Parent's signature _____

Instructions Log							
Date	Medication	Start Date	Finish Date	Dosage	Time	Parent's Signature	Administrator's Signature

Instructions Log							
Date	Medication	Start Date	Finish Date	Dosage	Time	Parent's Signature	Administrator's Signature

Medication Authorization and Instructions

Child's Name _____

Date _____

I grant permission to my childcare provider, _____
to administer the following medication to my child. I will therefore not hold my
childcare provider liable in the event of reactions or complications arising from
my child receiving this medication, once same is administered as per my
instructions below.

Parent's signature _____

Instructions Log							
Date	Medication	Start Date	Finish Date	Dosage	Time	Parent's Signature	Administrator's Signature

Instructions Log							
Date	Medication	Start Date	Finish Date	Dosage	Time	Parent's Signature	Administrator's Signature

Medication Authorization and Instructions

Child's Name _____

Date _____

I grant permission to my childcare provider, _____
to administer the following medication to my child. I will therefore not hold my
childcare provider liable in the event of reactions or complications arising from
my child receiving this medication, once same is administered as per my
instructions below.

Parent's signature _____

Instructions Log							
Date	Medication	Start Date	Finish Date	Dosage	Time	Parent's Signature	Administrator's Signature

Date	Medication	Start Date	Finish Date	Dosage	Time	Parent's Signature	Administrator's Signature

Medication Authorization and Instructions

Child's Name _____

Date _____

I grant permission to my childcare provider, _____
to administer the following medication to my child. I will therefore not hold my
childcare provider liable in the event of reactions or complications arising from
my child receiving this medication, once same is administered as per my
instructions below.

Parent's signature _____

Instructions Log							
Date	Medication	Start Date	Finish Date	Dosage	Time	Parent's Signature	Administrator's Signature

Date	Medication	Start Date	Finish Date	Dosage	Time	Parent's Signature	Administrator's Signature

Medication Authorization and Instructions

Child's Name _____

Date _____

I grant permission to my childcare provider, _____
to administer the following medication to my child. I will therefore not hold my childcare provider liable in the event of reactions or complications arising from my child receiving this medication, once same is administered as per my instructions below.

Parent's signature _____

Instructions Log							
Date	Medication	Start Date	Finish Date	Dosage	Time	Parent's Signature	Administrator's Signature

Date	Medication	Start Date	Finish Date	Dosage	Time	Parent's Signature	Administrator's Signature

Medication Authorization and Instructions

Child's Name _____

Date _____

I grant permission to my childcare provider, _____
to administer the following medication to my child. I will therefore not hold my
childcare provider liable in the event of reactions or complications arising from
my child receiving this medication, once same is administered as per my
instructions below.

Parent's signature _____

Instructions Log							
Date	Medication	Start Date	Finish Date	Dosage	Time	Parent's Signature	Administrator's Signature

		Instructions Log						
Date	Medication	Start Date	Finish Date	Dosage	Time	Parent's Signature	Administrator's Signature

Medication Authorization and Instructions

Child's Name _____

Date _____

I grant permission to my childcare provider, _____
to administer the following medication to my child. I will therefore not hold my childcare provider liable in the event of reactions or complications arising from my child receiving this medication, once same is administered as per my instructions below.

Parent's signature _____

Instructions Log							
Date	Medication	Start Date	Finish Date	Dosage	Time	Parent's Signature	Administrator's Signature

							Instructions Log		
Date	Medication	Start Date	Finish Date	Dosage	Time	Parent's Signature	Administrator's Signature

Medication Authorization and Instructions

Child's Name _____

Date _____

I grant permission to my childcare provider, _____
to administer the following medication to my child. I will therefore not hold my
childcare provider liable in the event of reactions or complications arising from
my child receiving this medication, once same is administered as per my
instructions below.

Parent's signature _____

Instructions Log							
Date	Medication	Start Date	Finish Date	Dosage	Time	Parent's Signature	Administrator's Signature

		Instructions Log						
Date	Medication	Start Date	Finish Date	Dosage	Time	Parent's Signature	Administrator's Signature

Medication Authorization and Instructions

Child's Name _____

Date _____

I grant permission to my childcare provider, _____
to administer the following medication to my child. I will therefore not hold my
childcare provider liable in the event of reactions or complications arising from
my child receiving this medication, once same is administered as per my
instructions below.

Parent's signature _____

Instructions Log							
Date	Medication	Start Date	Finish Date	Dosage	Time	Parent's Signature	Administrator's Signature

		Instructions Log						
Date	Medication	Start Date	Finish Date	Dosage	Time	Parent's Signature	Administrator's Signature

Medication Authorization and Instructions

Child's Name _____

Date _____

I grant permission to my childcare provider, _____
to administer the following medication to my child. I will therefore not hold my childcare provider liable in the event of reactions or complications arising from my child receiving this medication, once same is administered as per my instructions below.

Parent's signature _____

Instructions Log							
Date	Medication	Start Date	Finish Date	Dosage	Time	Parent's Signature	Administrator's Signature

Date	Medication	Start Date	Finish Date	Dosage	Time	Parent's Signature	Administrator's Signature

Instructions Log

Medication Authorization and Instructions

Child's Name _____

Date _____

I grant permission to my childcare provider, _____
to administer the following medication to my child. I will therefore not hold my childcare provider liable in the event of reactions or complications arising from my child receiving this medication, once same is administered as per my instructions below.

Parent's signature _____

Instructions Log							
Date	Medication	Start Date	Finish Date	Dosage	Time	Parent's Signature	Administrator's Signature

Date	Medication	Start Date	Finish Date	Dosage	Time	Parent's Signature	Administrator's Signature

Medication Authorization and Instructions

Child's Name _____

Date _____

I grant permission to my childcare provider, _____
to administer the following medication to my child. I will therefore not hold my childcare provider liable in the event of reactions or complications arising from my child receiving this medication, once same is administered as per my instructions below.

Parent's signature _____

Instructions Log							
Date	Medication	Start Date	Finish Date	Dosage	Time	Parent's Signature	Administrator's Signature

Date	Medication	Start Date	Finish Date	Dosage	Time	Parent's Signature	Administrator's Signature

**Instructions Log**.

Medication Authorization and Instructions

Child's Name _____

Date _____

I grant permission to my childcare provider, _____
to administer the following medication to my child. I will therefore not hold my childcare provider liable in the event of reactions or complications arising from my child receiving this medication, once same is administered as per my instructions below.

Parent's signature _____

Instructions Log							
Date	Medication	Start Date	Finish Date	Dosage	Time	Parent's Signature	Administrator's Signature

Date	Medication	Start Date	Finish Date	Dosage	Time	Parent's Signature	Administrator's Signature

Instructions Log

Medication Authorization and Instructions

Child's Name _____

Date _____

I grant permission to my childcare provider, _____
to administer the following medication to my child. I will therefore not hold my
childcare provider liable in the event of reactions or complications arising from
my child receiving this medication, once same is administered as per my
instructions below.

Parent's signature _____

Instructions Log							
Date	Medication	Start Date	Finish Date	Dosage	Time	Parent's Signature	Administrator's Signature

Date	Medication	Start Date	Finish Date	Dosage	Time	Parent's Signature	Administrator's Signature

Instructions Log

Medication Authorization and Instructions

Child's Name _____

Date _____

I grant permission to my childcare provider, _____
to administer the following medication to my child. I will therefore not hold my childcare provider liable in the event of reactions or complications arising from my child receiving this medication, once same is administered as per my instructions below.

Parent's signature _____

Instructions Log							
Date	Medication	Start Date	Finish Date	Dosage	Time	Parent's Signature	Administrator's Signature

Date	Medication	Start Date	Finish Date	Dosage	Time	Parent's Signature	Administrator's Signature

Instructions Log

Medication Authorization and Instructions

Child's Name _____

Date _____

I grant permission to my childcare provider, _____
to administer the following medication to my child. I will therefore not hold my childcare provider liable in the event of reactions or complications arising from my child receiving this medication, once same is administered as per my instructions below.

Parent's signature _____

Instructions Log							
Date	Medication	Start Date	Finish Date	Dosage	Time	Parent's Signature	Administrator's Signature

Date	Medication	Start Date	Finish Date	Dosage	Time	Parent's Signature	Administrator's Signature

Instructions Log

Medication Authorization and Instructions

Child's Name _____

Date _____

I grant permission to my childcare provider, _____
to administer the following medication to my child. I will therefore not hold my childcare provider liable in the event of reactions or complications arising from my child receiving this medication, once same is administered as per my instructions below.

Parent's signature _____

Instructions Log							
Date	Medication	Start Date	Finish Date	Dosage	Time	Parent's Signature	Administrator's Signature

Date	Medication	Start Date	Finish Date	Dosage	Time	Parent's Signature	Administrator's Signature

Medication Authorization and Instructions

Child's Name _____

Date _____

I grant permission to my childcare provider, _____
to administer the following medication to my child. I will therefore not hold my
childcare provider liable in the event of reactions or complications arising from
my child receiving this medication, once same is administered as per my
instructions below.

Parent's signature _____

Instructions Log							
Date	Medication	Start Date	Finish Date	Dosage	Time	Parent's Signature	Administrator's Signature

Date	Medication	Start Date	Finish Date	Dosage	Time	Parent's Signature	Administrator's Signature

Medication Authorization and Instructions

Child's Name _____

Date _____

I grant permission to my childcare provider, _____
to administer the following medication to my child. I will therefore not hold my childcare provider liable in the event of reactions or complications arising from my child receiving this medication, once same is administered as per my instructions below.

Parent's signature _____

Instructions Log							
Date	Medication	Start Date	Finish Date	Dosage	Time	Parent's Signature	Administrator's Signature

Date	Medication	Start Date	Finish Date	Dosage	Time	Parent's Signature	Administrator's Signature

Medication Authorization and Instructions

Child's Name _____

Date _____

I grant permission to my childcare provider, _____
to administer the following medication to my child. I will therefore not hold my childcare provider liable in the event of reactions or complications arising from my child receiving this medication, once same is administered as per my instructions below.

Parent's signature _____

Instructions Log							
Date	Medication	Start Date	Finish Date	Dosage	Time	Parent's Signature	Administrator's Signature

Instructions Log

Date	Medication	Start Date	Finish Date	Dosage	Time	Parent's Signature	Administrator's Signature

Medication Authorization and Instructions

Child's Name _____

Date _____

I grant permission to my childcare provider, _____
to administer the following medication to my child. I will therefore not hold my childcare provider liable in the event of reactions or complications arising from my child receiving this medication, once same is administered as per my instructions below.

Parent's signature _____

Instructions Log							
Date	Medication	Start Date	Finish Date	Dosage	Time	Parent's Signature	Administrator's Signature

				Instructions Log			
Date	Medication	Start Date	Finish Date	Dosage	Time	Parent's Signature	Administrator's Signature

www.ingramcontent.com/pod-product-compliance
Lightning Source LLC
Chambersburg PA
CBHW081156180526
45170CB00006B/2094